YOU ARE NOT ALONE

OVERCOMING ILLNESS AND STARTING A NEW ERA

BY CONNOR CARSON

A Four Clovers Publishing Publication
Four Clovers Publishing Registered Offices: Caldwell, NJ 07006

Library of Congress Control Number: 2026910178
Connor Carson
You Are Not Alone
ISBN: 979-8-9988858-6-0 (Print)
ISBN: 979-8-9988858-7-7(E-Pub)
Published in the United States of America
Book cover and original photography by Cole Carson
Inside design by Kristin Broek
Editing and creative design consultation by Taryn Lagonigro

In alignment with our commitment to inclusion, this book is set in an accessible font to support all readers and promote a more equitable reading experience.

While the author has made every effort to provide accurate information at the time of publication, neither the publisher nor the author assumes any responsibility for errors, or for changes that may occur after publication.

This book is creative nonfiction. The information and events in this book are the knowledge and memories of the authors and the writers within. The events have been expressed and written as remembered by the author. Certain names and identifying details have been omitted or changed to protect the privacy of the individuals.

Chapter List

Prologue

I was in my room, looking out the window, when an image from my head started playing out through it. I blinked with shock - I was looking back to the happy days. Watching myself running on the beach, having fun, “drinking”, and going on boat rides. It felt joyful looking back at those memories. It felt like a break from reality at the moment, to be able to look back and remember what I had felt like. Suddenly my mom opened the door to check on me and everything disappeared. I was back in reality, feeling sick and not knowing why.

SECTION 1: DAYLIGHT

Chapter 1
Life Before Illness

My story starts in the summer of 2021.
On a typical morning, I hear the birds sing or the cold air whistle and know it's time to wake up, but I take it slow. When I feel ready to get up, I go downstairs to relax and at some point to eat breakfast.

I start to feel the feelings of a jam in my body - it's time to get my speaker and dance like there's no tomorrow! I love to exercise and move my body in the morning, it helps me start my day. The sun is almost up for me to get ready for the day and do other things around the house.

Sometimes, on beautiful days, I will dance outside or take a walk and feel the air in my hair and have the feelings that something warm is about to bloom.

My family are members of a club in Harriman State Park called Thendara. We go swimming and kayaking on Lake Tiorati, which is close to our home. We walk down through the woods to get there in the summer. Going on a kayak, just listening to frogs croaking, looking up to the blue of the sky with the sun warming the water makes it so inviting to swim.

On the weekends, it's much busier when lots of members come. We have fires that we sit around, games we play and we all cook in the kitchen together. There are a lot of lovely people that listen to me and make me feel a part of the camp family.

Being outside really makes me feel alive. I felt the sun beaming on me with the fresh air just waking me up. No matter if there is snow on the ground or rain I try to get outside as much as I can.

At this time, I was working at a job I had since 2020 as a baker. During COVID times, we had to wear masks every day but it was good to be able to keep working.

I was able to develop a lot of skills at work. I am an excellent bread shaper, and spent time making dough for cookies and crackers - every day was different.

I loved socializing with my friends at lunch, talking about our weekends before heading back to work, not really talking much until the day has ended.

This was one of my first experiences with working, I learned a lot and was able to keep busy during that dark time of the pandemic.

We go on vacations to Cape Cod, MA, or to points on the Jersey Shore like Wildwood and Long Beach Island in the summer. I eat like crazy as the summer feels like a delicious time to eat without any restrictions, like having barbecues! There is nothing better than a juicy hamburger off the grill in the summertime and a hot dog with baked beans. And don't get me started with ice cream after a barbeque - it's very refreshing on a hot summer day!

That summer in particular, I was having an awesome time enjoying the summer, breathing in that warm fresh air. Running on the beach, having the time of my life with friends and family.

Life was great! I had freedom to go anywhere and eat whatever I wanted. I was feeling strong and satisfied. I wasn't limited, and I felt healthy and in shape.

I love being social, being outside, taking family or friends out for a meal, making smoothies, and looking at flowers in bloom.

When I go and take a walk I love looking at the plants blooming, seeing the blue sky, and feeling the sun just beaming on me. The reason why I love walking is because it gets me out of the house to move my body and stay in shape. It makes me feel awake and alive.

Having Down syndrome, I do have to see doctors regularly for low vision, cataracts, hypothyroid, heart defects, and minor ear issues. I've had some surgeries here and there, but everything has been under control and my health then was good.

Living with Down syndrome has many obstacles but good times as well. I have fun times with my family and they are so accepting of me as a part of the family.

Sometimes it is hard for me to not be able to do all of the same things as someone else. Some of my obstacles are when my family talks about a subject that I don't like, then I go in lock down and try not to leave the room. That's what I did when I was younger. Now I stay where I am and they see me in my own world and try to crack my shell and talk about something else. I wish sometimes that people could be a little bit more patient with people with disabilities. My brain takes a while for me to sync anything in, so sometimes I need some extra time. It can take me a longer time to get used to an environment and how to cope with it. Sometimes when situations are really busy it can feel a little chaotic in my brain. However,

I love being around so many different people, those with disabilities and those without!

When my birthday came that year, I turned twenty-one and I celebrated! I enjoyed being able to join in on what everyone else was doing. One of my cousins gave me a pack of non-alcoholic beer. Everybody kept telling me that I was legal, I could actually drink, but for health reasons, I don't drink alcohol. However, I love to drink non-alcoholic beers and non-alcoholic wine also. I love making exotic combinations with mocktails and ordering cool drinks at bars.

Being twenty-one was an enjoyable age, "drinking," having fun and dancing. That summer was one that I will never forget.

Chapter 2
The Unwelcomed Present

In the fall of 2022, the holidays rolled around. I love Thanksgiving, because it is a time to be with family. Spending this time with my family is my favorite part of the year. Christmas is my all-time favorite, because it feels magical seeing holiday lights and buying and wrapping gifts. It's really nice when my brother comes home from college - I enjoy his warmth and company.

I also have holiday traditions with my friends. We do a Friendsgiving which means we all bring something to eat and celebrate. On New Year's Eve we try to get together to celebrate the new year together by going to a nice restaurant.

I don't like Halloween, because it feels too scary and creepy for me. I dodge the creepyness by switching right to Christmas music. Dressing up is fun, just not the actual holiday itself.

That year, Thanksgiving weekend was very

exciting because we were seeing long lost relatives. They came over to our house and we sat around and chatted, feeling the love of getting to know each other again. We played games and laughed.

When our relatives left, I started to feel hot. I decided to take a test for COVID-19, and it was positive. We had no choice but to let my relatives know that they had been exposed, and some of them even wound up getting it too. Oh boy, it was an early Christmas gift for them. I went upstairs and went to bed emotionless. It also affected my sense of taste a little, and smell too.

I had COVID other times, but nothing like this before. To pass the time I mainly stayed in my room watching the iPad and mostly sleeping. If I had to, I would go downstairs to eat. I was so exhausted that I didn't do much to pass the time other than sleep.

My brother Cole had been home from college, and he was about to walk out the door to go back when he also started feeling sick. He also tested positive for COVID. Here we go again! If my mom was busy, I had to help my brother. He had such a high fever that we had to keep cold compresses on him at all times. I felt so bad for him. My mom, on the other hand, had fallen in the woods and broken a few ribs recently, so each time she had to take care of my brother and me, she would be trying to get up while yelling in pain.

You would think that would be enough, but guess what, somebody else gets COVID - my mom. Ugh, here we go again, the last person left. Boy, when I started developing COVID, I was looking out of the window in my bedroom, wondering when the lockdown was going to end. Then I had to be in isolation for ten more days, still looking at the same window, thinking when will my life begin again?

After COVID, I just kept getting sicker each day and what I called a malfunction came in January. There were a lot of days spent just looking out of the windows of my house and didn't know who I was, since something was igniting in my body. I was wondering when I would feel normal again.

In the end we believe that long covid from this illness is what caused my chronic medical issues. Now I will share that story with you.

SECTION 2: MIDNIGHT

Chapter 3
The Mystery Unfolding

Mystery Illness

Something was blossoming, and I didn't know what was happening. Every day was just the same on end with intense darkness and bitter cold. I was unable to get out of bed to take a shower. I was sliding down the steps to lie on the couch. It left me speechless. I wouldn't even get dressed, sitting in the dark with harsh light covering me, feeling chronic fatigue and dizziness. I was really lonely just being home by myself. It felt raw and painful.

The dark, lonely nights kept going without any answers. I was swallowing through pain. I remembered when I got up too fast from sitting, I would get lightheaded and dizzy every single time and didn't know why. With me getting dizzier by the minute and having trouble calming down, I would just stare into space with sorrow and darkness. I saw the rain from my window, and with the aches and confusion, I just lay in bed. My emotions changed quickly. I felt that the room was in a mini spin with everything going in circles, as every day was the same.

Going to work was the hardest. I couldn't leave the house, like there was a chain that couldn't be unlocked. I really missed my old self before any of this happened. Sometimes it hurts to have something that you've never experienced before. Mentally and physically, this was challenging.

My family had big question marks on their faces. My emotions changed from happiness to sadness and grief. Activities were hard because the dizziness came randomly. I wanted to move past it by forgetting it, but I knew that wasn't possible.

My bed felt like a boat floating off-stream. I didn't feel like myself. I didn't know who I was anymore. I let myself get into trouble. I wanted to get into trouble. With all of this happening, each night and day change, as some symptoms vary from day to day. The devil really was calling. No light, just darkness. Negative. Pulling me down in slow motion.

Sometime in January 2023, I started noticing that I was not hearing well, and mentioned that to my family. I was also having some occasional dizziness and pain around my ears. My mom wrote it off as a short-term issue that would resolve itself, so we did nothing! The feeling of being trapped and tortured. Looking out of the window with doors locked, with me visible inside, anybody except my support system would look inside. I was visible, but to others, they saw nothing, and I was in my own world. I continued to complain about the hearing loss, ringing in my ears, and then dizziness. Finally, everyone decided that my mom should pick up the phone. I'd better get to the doctor.

By now, it is mid-February. We went to my long-term ENT, where he conducted an audiology test. Through this we discovered that I had hearing loss in both ears, which was unusual and new for me. This concerned the doctor. He put me on steroids and sent us to a specialist. We got the appointment with the specialist while we were in Florida on vacation. We flew back to New Jersey and drove directly to a doctor at Mount Sinai in New York City. We got off the plane and went straight to the city in the snow - with no coats and no boots! We were freezing!! While at the specialist appointment, I had a horrible episode after my audiology test, a full-on vertigo attack. This was a shock - I had never experienced anything like it. I couldn't stand up, was shaking, burning hot, non-verbal and just staring blankly. The doctor was puzzled and concerned. He ordered a MRI, along with a tapering of the steroids and we rushed back home to get in our regular winter clothes, no closer to any answers.

Once the steroids were done and the MRI was completed, we returned to the specialist ENT to check in. There was still no improvement in the symptoms I was having and the MRI showed nothing. This doctor then recommended hearing aids and vestibular therapy. He still seemed puzzled by the loss of hearing that I was experiencing in both ears. Going to the doctor forced me to get out of my pajamas and actually have clothes on, but my clothes were very lowkey - I was feeling so annoyed that I just didn't care how I looked. Getting ready for the day, I felt like I was an outsider looking at my own life, feeling very bleak.

When we went to our first vestibular therapy appointment, the initial tests during the evaluation confused the therapists, because the findings were inconsistent. They wanted us to rule out anything more serious, so they asked us to go see a neurologist before returning to therapy.

Off to another doctor we went! The neurologist agreed that the MRI didn't show anything concerning. He wanted us to do an EEG (electroencephalogram) which records activity in the brain and tests for seizures. The one hour EEG was horrible, even though I was less dizzy from it than the other test. Then I had to wear a second EEG for three days and couldn't shower. The worst part was removing the wires on the last day - it felt like they used super glue to put them on. It took almost a week for the stickiness to go away.

From there, we went to another ENT, a neuro ophthalmologist, two different neurologists, had an MRI, a CT (computed tomography) scan, an EEG, an EKG (electrocardiogram) and for many other tests.

One day during this time, I was bloated and we weren't sure why - was it from the stress or from food? It was so bad that we decided to go to my primary care physician. She was concerned and sent me to the Emergency Room to get checked out. They sent me for a cat scan at that appointment, which showed nothing. It felt like we were there forever - we passed the time watching *Diners, Drive-Ins and Dives* for hours, our favorite show! We would even joke after that we wanted to go back to the ER to watch it, it was a nice distraction from what was going on. I had a blank stare episode while I was there and the doctors didn't know what to make of it. They weren't sure if they should keep me overnight or send me home, but luckily they sent me home because they didn't think it was serious enough to stay.

We were not done with our quest for answers yet. The neurologist had us do a MR angio, a non-invasive MRI that provides 3D images of blood vessels in your brain, helping doctors find blockages, narrowings and tears. The test showed some abnormalities, but the doctor felt like they were likely there from birth. Still no answers.

My life was shrinking around the unpredictability of it all. At times, I would zone out, stare, and shut down completely. I would get so dizzy that I couldn't stand and would collapse to the floor. I found myself crawling up and down stairs just to avoid falling. I was missing work.

When I was going through a dizzy spell, I would mainly call my family to help me to stay calm. They always told me to breathe, if a spell was getting more out of control and the intensity got harsh, they would keep on breathing with me over the phone. I think it was stressful both having these episodes and not knowing how it came.

During the summer, after eating breakfast, I would get dizzy but had no idea how it was set off. The heat would be intense and sometimes the heat in the summer would just come out of nowhere, which sometimes caused an episode. But mostly it was being anxious and scared was the main ingredient for a spell to develop. Sometimes even when I heard that my brother was coming home, I would get too excited and it would trigger a spell, which was not Cole's fault at all.

I was really lonely just being home by myself. I was swallowing through pain. I remember when I got up too fast from sitting, I would get lightheaded and dizzy every single time and didn't know why. With me getting dizzier by the minute and having trouble calming down, I would just stare into space with sorrow and darkness. I saw the rain from my window, and with the aches and confusion, I just lay in bed. My emotions changed quickly. I felt that the room was in a mini spin with everything going in circles, as every day was the same.

I just really missed being myself at this time of my life. Mainly being home, going nowhere for months felt full of despair and hopelessness. There was no way to get out of this, I felt like the windows had no light coming in, doors were locked, darkness was growing and the raw sadness and grief was settling in the house.

Even missing the sounds that were gone the house felt like a tunnel with everything echoing with sounds that I couldn't hear. A very dark, quiet place with nobody to talk to. I was trying to make every day count, but there was nowhere to go except going to doctor appointments.

I would try to figure out what I was going through, and getting a spell would have many reasons for how it could have gotten triggered. Since it was me going through this sometimes I would know what caused it, but some people didn't believe that it was the answer.

With spell after spell in the summer alongside with the heat I was convinced the heat would trigger an attack. Every single morning I would come down to watch *Switch at Birth* eating breakfast and just fall down. There was no way I would accept that guess it was not because of the show we would never know for sure. I knew there were other variables.

If I was lying on the floor with an attack I would've never come back up unless someone was there to pick me up. It felt so weird and felt like an outsider because, even in my own world. It was uncomfortable to be out in public. The only people that I knew what was going on were my support system. It was odd, I just wanted to give up and go home, but the only way to get better was to get out and do things - I didn't have a choice. I was laid back and when I was out trying to fit in I felt strange, like nobody would want to be with somebody who was uncanny and poorly dressed.

I really missed the smiles on everyone's faces, including mine. It felt like there was a chain on every single door locked shut, blinds closed, everything darkness was growing into a dark hole with such grief for my old life. I used to be so comfortable and mellow, but once I got sick, I didn't care how I dressed. I now had holes in my jeans and my style got very edgy. Every room felt like it was black and white.

It was hard at night time; being alone with the gravitational pull of grief for my old life. It felt like an alarm was flashing with all of these burning bright bold colors filling the rooms with caution. Each day when morning came, things got redder and bolder brighter than ever. It was very glaring!
The echoing of my screaming made the lights even brighter. A tornado was developing inside of my body with all these intense colors bouncing for months and didn't know how to deal with it.

This is the most extreme part of my life.

Keep Going: A Letter To My Sick Self

Through the years of being in the raw painful feelings, I wrote to myself about the hardest experience of my life. Now that I got better, I can go back and reread what I wrote. I wanted this to be something I can pull out of my pocket for encouragement to keep going when things get tough.

Dear Connor,

You are doing great trying to get through this. I know how you feel right now with the confusion and questions that you are asking yourself.

Going through a dark time is very tough. At some point there are going to be angels, they are going to be your support system. Try to make everyday count. You got this. Your mom was there to dry the tears after an attack. Her smile shined on your face. Now do the next right thing. All the stars are your support system shining down on you.

You finally have progress being made and you will love to see the man you became.

I am so proud of you for being brave and tolerating the mounds of vitamins - that takes a lot of effort.

You finally found it - your answers to everything relaxing when you need it and making everyday count.

Chapter 4
Diagnosis

In late April of 2023, we still had no real answers as we headed to a neuro ophthalmologist. At the end of the appointment, he said he didn't believe this was related to the eyes. We thought we were leaving another appointment with no answers. As he was leaving the room, he suggested that it could possibly be migraines and recommended we pick up the book *Migraines* by Oliver Sacks. My mom didn't think it would be any good for us because I never had a headache but she read it anyway and within the first 20 pages she saw all of my symptoms.

I never had headaches—never—which is why we didn't initially think what I was experiencing were migraines. For over a year, my symptoms showed up in other ways: diarrhea and abdominal pain, motion sickness, nausea, dizziness, hearing loss, autonomic issues, intermittent short-term hearing loss, ringing in my ears (tinnitus), deep fatigue—especially after episodes that were happening almost daily—pressure in my ears, and episodes of low blood pressure.

There might be light at the end of the tunnel! After reading the *Migraine* book, plus the research I had been doing on Meniere's Disease, we thought we were finally on to something. Symptoms for Meniere's disease include tinnitus, vertigo, headaches, pain, and pressure in the ear...many of the same things I was experiencing. We ran right to the ENT and told him what we thought it was and he agreed that he thought it was that and Meniere's disease combined. Finally, *finally* a diagnosis! Now can I get better?

The doctor told me right away to lower my sodium intake, which helps Meniere's, and take a tremendous amount of vitamins and medicine. Some worked, but some of them made things worse. We were told to go to vestibular therapy again. The therapists didn't know what I had, so they did lots of tests that took about two or three hours, and I had to suffer through it.

The red flags were waving as a signal that, oh no, things were not becoming controllable and much more severe. Therapy brought on the symptoms, and some days they would reach the next level. Not only was I dizzy at therapy, but also at home. I really had no break. Hearing aids were prescribed for me. This was the beginning of all the confusion. I would get dizzy if I got anxious, scared, and distressed. My doctor gave me motion sickness pills. They didn't help at all. They made me extra tired. This is the continuing of my mental lockdown. Doors locked, blinds closed. Darkness was kicking in more and more.

Vestibular Migraines

Vestibular migraines are not fun. Someone might get chronic headaches, blurry vision, bloating, light and noise sensitivity, nausea, motion sickness, and some similarities with Meniere's disease. Some days you can get one or the other or both on the same day. I went to therapy and thought it would help, but it worsened over time. I never experienced vomiting, only nausea.

Also, with the migraines, you can get these weird zoned out, spaced out moments with no verbal responses. This would make my mom really scared and distressed because she didn't know what was happening. Somehow, with my best knowledge, I was using American

Sign Language, trying to talk to my mom, but she had no clue what I was saying. Luckily she was able to understand some of the signs she taught me when I was younger.

The odd thing was that after these migraines, I had no memory of what happened. One time, Mom timed how long it lasted - ten minutes after my MRI was done - which was the longest one. She was trying to snap me out of it, but, with no response. At this point, she was almost in tears. The doctor didn't want to say, but said it anyway, "Should I call 911?" Luckily, at some point, I got out of it.

If you have either of these two conditions, I could tell you that many of you would want to be in a dark room, in the quiet, maybe sleeping a lot. I recommend no screens because that makes it more painful. Your ENT might put you on a diet, which I will explain more soon.

Chapter 5
Treatment

Having a diagnosis was only part of the solution. Now I have to get better! My doctors recommended a combination of medicines, vitamins, vestibular therapy and a major diet change while we figured out what worked for me to recover.

Vestibular Therapy

One day at therapy, the lights were bouncing with my eyes getting much blurrier by the minute. The first step of healing went terribly wrong. As the people were so kind and helpful, trying to pull me up as my ears wanted to pull me down, like gravity slamming me into the ground. I was also trying to catch my breath. All of my symptoms felt like they came alive in therapy. My eyes felt like I was looking through a kaleidoscope with harsh lights that couldn't see clearly. I was lying on a hard, wobbly ground with crazy tinnitus like a whistle in my ear! I just lost myself.

Oh, vestibular therapy! That was tough. One day, when everything was still mysterious, we went to physical therapy to be tested for a variety of things. The therapists were so nice, but they basically had to induce the symptoms and teach me how to cope with them. As I got tossed and turned during the testing, we thought it would help, but it actually made things worse.

Once we had my diagnosis, we had to go back to therapy. The therapist understood more about my symptoms when they knew I had vestibular migraines and when they researched Meniere's disease. The appointments were almost daily for several weeks. A typical therapy appointment would start with my vitals being taken. Then they would have me focus on things, like doing a puzzle or matching activities. Some days this was easy and some days my eyes were so foggy that I couldn't do it. The appointments were only an hour long but it felt like it went on forever! Even the ride to and from the appointment made me dizzy with motion sickness. This was a horrible few weeks. It did not work, and every visit was so difficult and scary! After a month or so, we stopped the vestibular therapy.

It was just a hell of a mess. Dizziness, blurry vision, tinnitus and also trying to catch my breath. Now I knew I was in trouble and creeping into danger! Screaming with my eyes as things got blurrier by the minute. The first step of healing felt like it wasn't going right at all.

Therapy was bringing on a progression of hearing loss. I was scared, and I reached out to my brother to ask him an important question. "I know that you are busy with work, but is there any way you could learn sign language?" So he thought about it, and he said yes. Each Monday night was an ASL (American Sign Language) lesson. His girlfriend also learned. They were patient and had some late nights working on ASL lessons together. He is an awesome brother. I am so proud he is my brother and feel very fortunate.

Diet

As part of trying to understand and manage my symptoms, my doctor put me on a strict migraine elimination diet. He also gave me some new medicines and told me to make sure I stayed hydrated as much as possible. He gave my mom and I all of the information about the new diet, and right away we got busy getting the ingredients and cooking only from the diet. It was incredibly hard, incredibly strict and *incredibly no fun at all*!

The neurologist had also put me on some medicine so between the two doctors I was on a few different pills everyday. We assumed that they were working in conjunction with the diet. At first, I didn't fully grasp how extensive the diet would be. It required cutting out foods known to be high in glutamates, MSG, tyramine, and certain additives—ingredients that can overstimulate the nervous system and trigger vestibular symptoms in some people.

Many of these ingredients are hidden in everyday foods under names like "natural flavors," yeast extracts, hydrolyzed proteins, or store-bought broths, making it far more complicated than simply avoiding obvious junk food (which I didn't normally eat anyway).

Beyond just additives, the list of foods to avoid was long and, at times, discouraging. Caffeine, chocolate, processed meats, aged cheeses, fermented foods, certain fruits, soy products, nuts, and even leftovers older than a few days were off-limits during the elimination phase. Foods I once ate without a second thought—

hot dogs at a barbecue, a piece of chocolate, or citrus fruits in the morning—were suddenly potential triggers. Eating became less about enjoyment and more about vigilance, reading labels, and fear of setting off another episode.

The goal of the diet was never meant to be permanent. It was designed as a temporary reset—something to follow until my symptoms were better controlled, with the hope of slowly reintroducing foods over time. Still, during that period, it changed how I moved through the world. I had to be very strict, otherwise the symptoms would return. Meals were smaller, safer, and stripped of spontaneity. While the diet did help bring clarity to my diagnosis and symptoms, it also highlighted how deeply illness can impact daily life—not just physically, but emotionally and socially as well.

The misery my mom must have had cooking not only for the family, but also for my brother and me, because we both couldn't have nuts, since that was one of the foods that was on the list I couldn't eat. It was horrific! I felt so bad for mom doing extra work; it was made with extra love and hard work. I just wanted to be like everyone else. One night I talked to my brother's girlfriend, crying because I didn't feel the same way, and jealous that everyone was eating the stuff that I couldn't eat. I just wanted to be myself again.

The sky was full with very sharp dynamic colors. The sun was glowing; beating on me with the rays making me dizzy. Things got crazier and now it started to rain. This time the rain felt like it was coming down with rainbow colors splashing down - like the sky was blending the colors. We were so confused why this was happening. The world was becoming colorful and I was in the center of it. With the heat this would make me feel nasty and violent on the inside. Leaving attacks with a feeling of being lightheaded. I had no clue why I was having episodes feeling like I was having a fever with sweat dripping making the summer more cruel. It really got to me in blinding, looking in the sky with it looking like a light blue.

When I was on the diet there were a lot of events happening that summer and I couldn't participate in them because the food that anybody served was out of the diet range. I had to bring my own food with me wherever I went. It was incredibly difficult and frustrating to stick to this. Birthday parties, barbeques, and just going out for dinners were a challenge. The table was really turning on me. I just wanted to roll my eyes with annoyance. That summer was so restricted it just didn't feel like a normal summer like the olden days. I couldn't "drink" or eat my favorite foods and was not feeling like myself.

One of my doctors put me on lots of different pills. More than you can even imagine, mounds of vitamins. They had some effect on me, not strong enough to actually make my symptoms disappear. A new nightmare was developing. And a big twist came with the diet; it was endless! We had to be extremely careful about what I was eating; one screw-up would make the next day into a mess of dizziness, tinnitus, and some of the migraine symptoms.

But I kept going, and suddenly one time on vacation, I realized I wasn't getting any symptoms at all from slipping from the diet. When I got home. I told mom that everything I ate on vacation was off the diet and I didn't get any symptoms. Mom did not believe me at first but we went back to the ENT and they said that a mixture of meds was working! Could I finally stop this horrible diet?!

One of my doctors told us that I could stop

the diet, so we ripped it up and burned it into flames.

The diet was outrageous and such a nightmare. We decided to never think about it again and get off of it! I still have to be a little bit careful and can't overdo it in certain areas otherwise I will feel some symptoms, but I could mostly eat regularly.

When we stopped it, boy did I celebrate big time! One day when I was working at the bakery, the table was filled with food that I ate like no tomorrow. When I got home, I felt like I was about to be sick - but just from eating too much, not from what I ate.

Since the day we burned the paper of the diet and ripped it into a million pieces, eating regularly again became a new normal. It felt amazing, and truly it was the help of my supporters along the way who made this possible for me to have the life that I had before.

I was getting exhausted from all of this and wanted to get out of this extreme summer. So my brother saw me and asked if I wanted to go somewhere to breathe. I said yes. We got in the car and we drove miles and miles. At the beginning of the ride I felt like I was hearing my screaming in my head, then it got gradually softer and eventually it disappeared. After that I fell asleep. While I was asleep Cole picked up his girlfriend and my mom and decided to go to Grace Farms to have a fun night out.

With all of the chaos I slept some more and when my eyes opened my brother was there to make sure that I was ok. Everything became calmer after that.

SECTION 3: GOLDEN HOUR

Chapter 6
Support

The day I lost my memory

On a cold fall night, on the way to dinner after a hard day, I took two migraine pills instead of one. We were hoping that doubling the medicine would mask my symptoms, but we were completely wrong. Looking out of the car window, the sun was setting, and my emotions fell to zero. I felt the world had fallen. My thoughts were holding back my words, they kept echoing in my head and I couldn't get them out of my mouth.

When my brother came to my car door, I felt like I saw sparkles in his eyes. The traffic lights were a blur behind him. Cole knew that something was wrong with me and that the cold air would help. My future was gradually looking brighter.

My brother started using American Sign

Language (ASL) to talk to me and I was able to respond. I couldn't believe that my brother and I were signing together in ASL. Even though my memory was wiped, I still knew how to sign! With all of the lessons that we did, he did the best job that night, talking with his hands. It felt so magical.

When I snapped out of it, my words came back, and my feelings popped out again. For that night, ASL unlocked the path.Then we held hands and went into the restaurant to have our dinner.

On the way home from dinner, we talked about how we had thought if I took two migraine pills that it would help my symptoms. We were wrong! My mom, my brother and I agreed that we would not try that again.

It was really hard to push through this hard time in my life. It was very challenging in a way that I couldn't do this alone. Being home alone was also not helping. I needed to be with my family or friends to have company. In the peak of my dizzy episodes, where things were getting worse and worse, I had to text and ask my grandma or my aunt to come over and stay with me. It was helpful to have them there because if I was doing chores around the house and all of a sudden I got a big vertigo attack they could help me up.

I needed the help from everyone for this tremendous challenging illness that made me not myself. No matter if it was a test that I had to do at home or just a normal day with dizzy spells, there was somebody who came over to help me to lift me up. Their help made the episode go away faster. Without the support system I had, I think this whole time would have lasted a lot longer. But we said heck no and made sure that it would take less time and that it went in the right direction.

There were many ways that my family supported me during this time. Everyone brought their smiles and bright faces back in my life every time they came over - it felt like they would have this mini spark of color that would come out of them. My friends were really supportive as well. My friend Russ, who I have known since middle school, even called me every night to make sure that I was okay.

Before we got my diagnosis, we were confused and scared at the same time because we had no clue what was happening. It kept happening again and again at the same place and when they were with me.

Once I was healed, I realized that it was all of this support that got me through it. It was then that I wanted to understand their experience of watching me go through this. I knew what it felt like to be scared, confused and frustrated. While I was experiencing the symptoms, they were experiencing uncertainty too. They were watching, waiting, worrying, and trying to be strong for me. I began to wonder what those days had felt like for them through their eyes.

My brother Cole was very close to the process, even from afar. When he saw it for the first time he understood perspective on what I was going through—and what it was like to watch it all unfold from the outside.

He told me that the first time he realized something was really wrong was through phone calls, when Mom and I tried to explain what was happening. But the first time he witnessed an episode in person was when he was home and I had a non-alcoholic drink, which may have made me dizzy. Seeing it up close scared him. He wasn't at home, he didn't know how to help, and that helplessness stayed with him. The only times that he knew what I was going through was when he came home. Cole was helpful when he was home but it was much harder to help over the phone.

For Cole, it became harder just to hang out the way we used to. So much of our time together was overshadowed by the fear that I might have another episode, and I wasn't really my fun, relaxed self anymore. He had never heard of Ménière's disease before, but he later learned that our great-grandmother had it too, which somehow made it feel both heavier and more real.

The ASL lessons were especially important to him. He wanted to be able to communicate with me if my hearing worsened, but he also admitted that he hated the fact that we even had to worry about that. Still, he tried—though he laughs now remembering how bad he actually was at learning sign language.

He told me he started to notice real improvement when I eventually got off the restrictive diet. Our interactions began to feel normal again, without everything being so fixated on my symptoms. When I would have an episode, he would remind me to breathe and would hug me, grounding me in a way that words couldn't.

Family gatherings weren't hard for him to navigate or adjust for—he was always happy to help—but he admitted that he spent much of that time quietly hoping I wouldn't have an episode.

One of his strongest memories was the first time he saw me have an episode in public — going down the stairs at the T station in Boston. I got dizzy, had to sit down, and my eyes started rolling. It was the first time he experienced it fully, and it stayed with him. We tried everything back then—fans, hydration, so many ideas—just trying to get through it.

And then there are the lighter memories, the ones that came after. He remembers a moment when things had settled and we were able to have a beer together again, though neither of us can remember where we were. That feels fitting somehow. Healing didn't arrive all at once, but it arrived quietly, in moments like that.

Maria, my brother's girlfriend, told me what it was like for her to witness my experience from a distance.

She told me how hard and scary it was to watch me go through everything while being so far away, wanting to help but not knowing how. Not being physically present made the helplessness even heavier. She shared that one of the hardest parts was watching pieces of who

I was slowly disappear—my ability to eat good food, my carefree attitude, and the ease I once moved through life. Instead, so much of my energy was spent worrying about when the next episode might happen.

Maria had heard of vestibular migraines and Ménière's disease before, but admitted she didn't fully understand them at the time. Like so many of us, she learned as we went.

She noticed a real shift when I was finally able to eat normally again and began gaining weight back. That's when she saw parts of me return—more present, more relaxed, more like myself. During the worst spells, she focused on helping me stay calm and safe, reminding me again and again that I was okay, that I was safe, and that it would pass.

One of her favorite memories came after I started recovering. She laughs now when she talks about how excited I was over something so simple—hot dogs! We didn't celebrate with anything big. The celebration was just being back to normal, and that was more than enough.

My Uncle Tom noticed when everything was unfolding. He told me that he knew something was wrong almost immediately because I wasn't my usual *"Mr. Funny"*. I stopped joking the way I normally do, and I couldn't eat many of the foods I've always loved. That change made him sad—not just because of the food, but because humor has always been such a big part of who I am.

He shared how hard it was to watch both me and my mom struggle to figure out what was happening. The uncertainty was heavy, and there were no clear answers for a long time. Uncle Tom had heard of Ménière's disease before, but vestibular migraines were new to him. He began to notice improvement when we started locking in on a diagnosis. Slowly, I started to come back—joking more, laughing again, feeling more like myself. He especially noticed the difference once I could eat the foods we love again, those familiar meals that always made family time feel normal.

What he remembers most is how good it felt simply to be together as a family—enjoying each other's company with less worry hanging over us. Those moments of normalcy mattered more than we realized at the time.

My Aunt Lynn learned about what was happening with me through my mom.

She told me there is nothing harder than watching someone you love deal with medical issues. One of the things she missed most was my usual joyful self—the lightness and ease that had always been part of who I was. Although she had heard of these illnesses before, that didn't make it any easier to see them affect someone so close to her.

Aunt Lynn noticed improvement when I began to seem more like myself again. During spells, she encouraged me to breathe and relax, helping me stay grounded when things felt overwhelming. She shared that it was never difficult for her to accommodate me at family events—I was doing the best I could, and she was always willing to meet me where I was.

She doesn't remember a specific moment when everything turned around, or any big celebration when it was over. But maybe that's because healing didn't arrive all at once. It came quietly, in small shifts, until one day things simply felt more normal again.

My mom was truly the one who was in the thick of it more than anyone. She told me she first knew something was really wrong when I kept saying, over and over, "I can't hear," and "I'm dizzy." It had been going on for about a month before she finally said she really listened in a different way. That's when it hit her that this wasn't just a phase or something small.

When I asked her how it made her feel when I was sick, she didn't hesitate. She said it was horrible. She hated every minute of it. She said I was miserable, and she felt helpless because she couldn't fix it. That was hard to hear, but also important.

She told me she missed the normal stuff. She missed talking about regular, everyday things instead of dizziness, hearing problems, doctor's appointments, and food. She missed just living with me without everything revolving around symptoms. I never really thought about how much that changed her life too.

I asked her if she had ever heard of vestibular migraine or Meniere's disease before all this. She said she knew about Meniere's because her grandma had it. She had heard the term vestibular migraine before, but she didn't really know what it meant. She also said she wished we had read the migraine book earlier. If we had those clues sooner, she thinks it could have changed a lot.

When I asked when she noticed I was starting to feel better, she said she saw a little improvement when we started what she calls "the stupid diet," and then bigger improvement when the new medication kicked in. That's when she finally felt hopeful.

I asked her what she would say to encourage me during a bad spell. She laughed and said there wasn't much any of us could say except "relax and breathe." As boring as that sounds, she said those were the only tools we had.

I also asked if it was hard accommodating me at family events. She said yes — it stunk! She had to plan my food in advance, and she had already been doing that for years for my brother because of his food allergies. She told me she remembers that summer in Cape Cod when she had to cook one special meal for him, one special meal for me, and then something else for everyone else — while everyone was out romping in the sand. She said that part was exhausting.

When I asked about a funny memory, she said the EEG with the wires glued to my head for three days was kind of funny — but not really. And she remembered all the hours in the emergency room, when I had so many symptoms and we were all scared, but we tried to laugh anyway. We watched our favorite shows and called Cole, trying to make something normal out of something that definitely wasn't.

Hearing her side made me realize something I hadn't fully understood before: while I was fighting what was happening inside my body, my family was fighting it too — just in a different way.

CHAPTER 7

Healing

The bare trees were making a creaking sound and made everything desolate quiet.

The memories would come often. There was no way to cope with it. Everywhere in mirrors and windows would just keep reminding me about those lovely days.

Those blinds that we closed for the three months were starting to have a slight opening and I couldn't believe winter snow was still on the ground and the winter wind was howling.

This time around still having mental problems and still having vertigo attacks. Most of the time thinking about those memories would get into my head.

Once I was getting better, sometimes a slight thought would bring me down, and it would come in flashes - like old memories or wishful thoughts. Even though I was starting to feel better, the healing was taking a while. Sometimes the flashes would have feelings that come along with them. The days when I get these feelings, they keep flashing back over and over. They would just ruin my day. Sometimes, calling my family was the best thing for me to get my feelings out.

These memories were setting me back.
I felt aches and pains. It felt annoying and exhausting. Getting slammed again and again. I couldn't handle it anymore. The devil followed me into this feeling of hopelessness. It felt like depression replaced some of my symptoms.

Pretty much every time, if I had a slight thought that brought me down, I would also get dizzy, as worrying and crying actually made things worse. Even having crazy thoughts and lots of distress made me get dizzier.

A big part of having these memories really changed me in a large way. Sometimes the memories would affect me all day, and it would frustrate me that everyone thought the answer would be to call my mom. She thought that she had to fix whatever I was feeling...but I felt like she had already been through enough. I refused to have that happen because I planned to have phone calls if I was home alone, not have my mom come to save the day just because I had feelings for that day.

I didn't feel like myself at all. Trying to go out and have a normal day with a friend and in the car looking out of the window still having these memories with no emotions other than dizziness. Every car ride I was on, most of the time I would feel motion sickness and nausea. Trapped in the house because it was too cold or I was having spots of dizziness. I wanted it to be concealed and trying not to feel it, but sometimes it would pop out of nowhere. I was trying to enjoy things but I just felt numb and sad. I was starting to feel better, but it felt bittersweet, because I missed my old life.

I was starting to have better days. Trying to get out as much as I can. Gravity was really pulling me. Having more fun days as it made my day seeing smiling faces again. Those days were fun but sometimes turned into migraine dizzy days. This time at least we knew what was wrong and I knew how to cope with it by laying down with white noise to help me to relax during an episode.

After Diet

When I was done with all of my severe symptoms, I celebrated big time—kept having what I wanted with no problem, including having my non-alcoholic beers. When we tore up the paper of the diet, we celebrated. I screamed in excitement that after three months on the diet, I was done. Finally being free and going out feels awesome. It feels great to have no more problems.

I told myself that I would never have chocolate again because I couldn't have it when I was on the diet, but I kinda slipped and started to have it again. I lost nine pounds from the diet, and all of my pants fell off!! I guess it was ok that I slipped, I needed my pants to fit again! Finally, feeling like a man going to a bar and having non-alcoholic beers was amazing. Going to restaurants with friends and family was great with no limitations. Thanksgiving and Christmas got a little crazier than normal, and I was eating nonstop. I really decked the halls and jingled to a new life.

I will always have Meniere's, but I don't have to worry about being on a diet. You need to eat some things in moderation. Too much salt and chocolate is not good, so be careful that you don't eat it all at once, but you can slip up once in a while.

A Healed Holiday

Looking out of the window with snow falling and sparkles as magic was in the air it's now the time to be cozy by the fire. Stockings hung up with care as the holidays are blowing in. In our house with static warm lights hanging on the tree. Decorating and drinking hot chocolate with wrapping gifts. In our pj's listening to the crackling fire.

During the holiday season, especially Thanksgiving, I ate a lot more than I did in previous years.

Now Christmas was coming, and there was more food to eat! I couldn't believe that my supportive elves made it possible to surround the room with laughter and joy and have more fun than I have had in a long time.

That Christmas, I was waiting for a chair to pull in and enjoy a meal. I felt the fun that I hadn't had for three months. No more painful memories. All of the joyful memories won.

My Christmas list was being with my family, walking in the snow and hearing it crunch, seeing holiday lights with the snow falling from the sky, which felt therapeutic, and seeing our breath in the winter air.

Life Coach

I felt like I was living through a fog, even my face looking puzzled most of the time. One day, a human figure appeared in the distance. While she was walking to my door, her sunrays were bouncing off the walls, almost like lifting the mist I was living within. She waved her magic wand, and one day I had no more symptoms. I was free.

Even with all of the progress that I was making, like being off the diet and starting to work again, I was still in a mental fog. I didn't know when this illness was going to end. It felt like when I was looking out the window, everything appeared mysterious. I was still going through such a rough time.

My mom introduced me to a life coach named Cherlyn because we were desperate to find someone to help me. We started to have weekly sessions. Sometimes, before our sessions, I would get dizzy or tense, and she would make me feel looser. She reminded me of my life before any of this happened. Now Cherlyn and I go to cafes and stores and get to enjoy everyday life. I love her so much. She really changed my emotions and outlook.

Cherlyn wanted me to reflect on everything we worked on together—and what really helped me through the hardest moments.

When I asked her which exercises made the biggest difference, she smiled and said, "All of them." But some stood out more than others. Breathing was huge for me. Pausing. Exhaling slowly. That became one of my favorites. When things felt out of control, I could always come back to my breath. Humming helped too. Sighing. Even smiling—just slightly—could shift something in my body.

We practiced focusing techniques, like grounding myself in nature. I'll never forget going outside to look at the butterflies on the butterfly bush. That moment reminded me that the world was still beautiful, even when I didn't feel well.

One of the most important things she taught me was this: nothing is forever. Episodes aren't forever. Fear isn't forever. Even bad days aren't forever. Knowing I was going to be okay—even when I didn't fully believe it yet—became something I could hold onto.

We did guided meditations where I would scan my body from head to toe, noticing each part and allowing myself to relax. I still go back to that practice whenever I'm not feeling well. It's like a reset button.

She also taught me the 5-4-3-2-1 method—using my senses to bring myself back to the present moment. Five things I can see. Four I can feel. Three I can hear. Two I can smell. One I can taste. That redirection really helped when my mind wanted to spiral.

Another lesson that stuck with me was being less resistant and more willing to go with the flow. That was a favorite of mine. Fighting what was happening only made it worse. When I stopped resisting and started accepting, even just a little, things felt lighter.

Making the best of any situation was harder for me. But that's where I started to feel grateful for the support around me. When Cherlyn walked into a session, it sometimes felt like the fog was lifting. She helped me remember the simple things that made me feel good—hot chocolate, music, small joys. Those little things mattered.

When I asked her what changes she saw in me from the beginning until now, she said she saw confidence. She saw me using the tools to take care of myself, becoming more independent, trusting myself more. She said I seemed empowered and self-reliant. Hearing that meant a lot to me.

When I asked what she learned from working with me, her answer surprised me. She said she learned that being happy is about being yourself—and that I was always myself. She told me she watched me sing, dance, and enjoy simple things like Taylor Swift and hot chocolate. She said my joy reminded her how powerful the little things in life can be.

Her advice to anyone going through something hard is simple: get to know yourself by listening to your body. Be still. Don't be afraid of what you're feeling. Let your feelings rise up and tell you what you need—and then give yourself what you need.

Take a nap. Go for a walk. Dance. Sing. Eat something healthy. Be creative. Use what you're going through to grow.
She told me she uses me as an example. She said I chose to do everything I could to help myself- including learning sign language. And now I'm writing this book to make sense of what happened and hopefully help someone else.

That's when I realized something important. Healing isn't just about getting better. It's about learning how to be with yourself in a new way.

And I hope all of these practices have helped me. I think they have.

Well-Being

If you are going through something like this, the best thing you can do is be outside and close your screens. If you are still going through vertigo, it might be harder to urge yourself to get out and enjoy the fresh air.

Sometimes it can be frustrating to go out if you feel dizzy and don't feel safe, but at least try. My favorite way to relax is to meditate. It's good for your mind and body. This helps to reset and will calm down your dizziness. This is one way to manage your symptoms.

It blows my mind that I came from having symptoms every day to nothing. You still need to remember to breathe and remind yourself that it will pass. Don't let the devil pull you down. Let the angel guide you in the other direction. You have to listen to your inner self.

How music changed my life

One of the most powerful tools to help me feel better was music. It changed my life. You can't control what's happening in this world, but music can help you to keep calm, and it can also make you dance! It helped me to be more positive and happier, and changed my emotions from scared to nothing. I promised myself to tune out the fear.

It helps your mental health to listen to music. Cancel out watching reels on social media, as that creates distress. Just *shake it off* when stress is getting to you!

During my rough time, I would turn on relaxing music to calm down. After I got much better, sometimes I would get scared about other things, and music would help. Taylor Swift's music specifically got into my head and she helped me mentally, big time!

Believing the positive made me brighter and brighter every day. It's just amazing how I became a Swiftie. Music in general is good for you. It helps to have a positive attitude, and it's a great way to start your day.

Love and Magic

One summer day, I was driving with my mom to Cape Cod with the wind in my hair.

The sun was about to set with pink clouds in the sky. On the horizon of the beach, and the lip of the ocean, something was waiting for me, but I did not know what it was. The pink clouds were dreamy, and they got me thinking as it got darker and darker as the sun set.

Finally, I got to Cape Cod and had a better night's sleep there in a house with my family. I was wondering what was finally going to be my cure. The mystery of my healing was still unknown until the day after.

The next day, it was very hot in Cape Cod. After the boat ride, we were cooking dinner for a big crowd, and we were talking about the diet and why I couldn't have certain foods. My cousin heard us talking, came in, and told me that the cure was love, and kissed me on the head.

The wind from the beach and the water from the ocean just blew and washed everything away, and that summer, the cure was all about love. And my family showed me great examples of how they could define fun; they also brought light to my life. My family can't get any closer than we already are. We can get closer and closer as much as we want.

Along with the lovable support, the meds were also magical, helping me like no tomorrow. They were a handful, but we did it. We think that there was a mixture of meds that helped me. I just want to say thank you to the entire family for their generosity, for saving me and making me the great man that I am today.

Don't pull back

My emotions changed dramatically. My old self was becoming a new self. From the exhaustion of taking medications as I was shifting from sadness and scared. To happiness and bravery. The diet after being shattered and burned into flames, including the mounds of meds that didn't work. I am never ever going back, like ever!

After going through a chronic disease that affected your life, a year later, you still think about those tragic days. Sometimes this feeling comes back and gives you these thoughts in your head. You might worry that you will feel like that again, which is very normal to feel.

You have to lift yourself and call the doctor if

your illness is still ongoing, or if it has been resolved, just go outside to feel the satisfaction and accomplishments you've achieved.

Tell yourself, "I am doing everything I can to pull it together and go to work or school and have a great day!" The best way is not to have the feelings that you had a year ago. The survivors who went through it, we are never ever ever going through the hell of that again! Just accept your new reality, and also the people who surround you. A new era is about to transform.

EPILOGUE
A New Era

One morning I heard and saw a big slash of lightning and thunder. I ran outside and everything bloomed and the sky was clear and blue. Life felt amazing. I could feel the wind through me. Finally, I can choose my own happiness.

There was a door that would bring me to Florida. Once I got there, I was listening to the acoustics and unpacking. I closed the dresser, leaving my old self behind, starting a new me.

Feeling the tropical breeze over the beach, breathing in the air. I was enjoying the beach and getting a tan. One night I went out for dinner at a bar. On the way home my family was on a balcony with fireworks shooting out of their bodies - as I was getting closer my spark in me got bigger and bigger. My family and I saw them to celebrate a brighter future.

To stay healthy these days, I dance in the morning and am active throughout the day. I love being outside - when the sun beats on me it soaks me with energy that makes me feel much more awake. Being outside just makes me feel that I have accomplished something throughout the day. I feel much more awake when I get out to listen to music or take a walk. As far as my diet, I still need to make sure not to eat too much chocolate. When I feel like I need to calm down or just have a slight reset, meditation comes into play and helps to remind me I am not going back.

Sometimes when I get a head cold, seasonal allergies or am in enough elevation to make my ears click, migrane or Meniere's symptoms trigger, which is annoying. Allergies, a cold or high elevation cause pressure in my ears and head, which often means I will feel dizzy the next day. One time, I was even rock climbing with my brother when I got dizzy...what bad timing! Now when I get these symptoms it's easy to know how to handle it.
Of course I need to be patient, because time tells when it's going to end, I don't get to control how much time. Tinnitus and being unstable not being able to do much is normal. For me, managing my symptoms is to take a ten minute nap to reset my body because vertigo takes a lot out of you.

When I get dizzy, I know how to angle my body and sit when it happens. I also can do my breathing exercises to help myself feel better. If it happens with my family now I know to go outside to get some air and come back in when I am ready. Now I can deal with it myself and don't really need anybody to comfort me unless it comes more intensely. We will knock on wood to make sure the symptoms will never come back in a big way (or ever!).

I feel very lucky that I have a community that I love being around. I am a social butterfly and love to talk forever! I feel very lucky that I thrive with Down Syndrome. There are a lot of things that my family did for me that make me feel lucky.

I am most proud that I got through this whole situation. With my family's help, it was somewhat easier to get through it together. It is more fun to be frustrated together than alone. The experience was hard and difficult but, there is a bright side to it, which was an appreciation for life.

In the fall of 2026, I am starting college and am really looking forward to that. I am most excited for this book to come out and get the word out to help other people. Life is treating me so much better, like feeling bright and happier. It would be really exciting if I could be famous one day! I am looking forward to future opportunities. My dream is that this book it's going to be a good example for others. For the future, my goals are to learn new things and become smarter and hope to be able to have more opportunities for work and grow as an author.

Starting a new era is also exciting and nerve racking - every time you shift new things it will always be scary, but there can be a bright side. I am excited about the future!

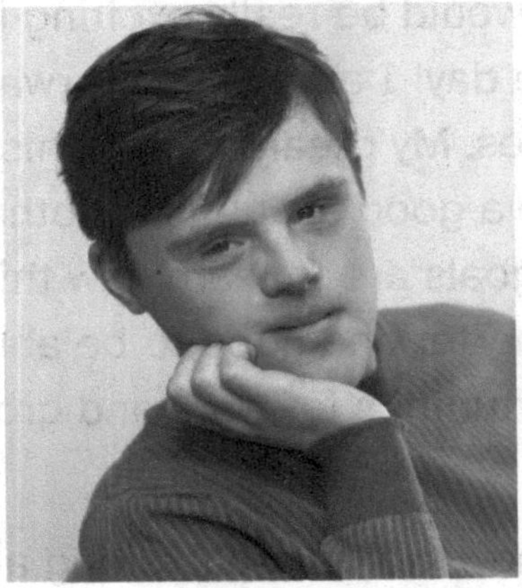

About the Author

Connor Carson was born with Down syndrome and grew up in northern New Jersey with his family. His career so far has included volunteering as a baker for a non-profit bakery and also working at a local cafe. He enjoys learning new languages including ASL, German, French and Spanish, playing the ukulele, being with friends, and playing lots of sports. Connor loves music, counting himself as a big Swiftie. *You Are Not Alone* is Connor's first book, which he was inspired to write after a long journey with chronic illness, to help others going through a similar experience. Connor is looking forward to growing as an author and writing more in the future!

Acknowledgements

I would love to thank Peg for helping me to start this journey to make this book come alive. I am pretty sure that mom told you everything that I was going through, which was easier to understand where I was going with the storylines.

To my mom for helping to make this book happen and for all the support while I was going through this dark time. I appreciate all the patience you had to have along the way. I am grateful I had you to lean on.

And to my brother Cole for your help with the photography and book cover design - your designs are outstanding. Thank you so much for helping me with this journey, especially with all the hugs and reminding me that it would pass.

And to all of my family for supporting me and guiding me, which led to me making this book. You put me in a path of happiness and I am so grateful for that. Thank you for your interviews to make this book more robust and give me your side of what you saw. That makes me feel like this work mattered and I'm thankful. Thank you for your help completing our mission together. Hand in hand makes everyday count!

www.ingramcontent.com/pod-product-compliance
Lightning Source LLC
LaVergne TN
LVHW040521210926
848480LV00007BA/1551